GJ II Ashwood was born in a wee town (city) called Belfast, N. Ireland, in the spring of 1981. Humble & working class beginnings, a childhood with guidance and plenty of craic with his parents, siblings and extended family, much in the northern irish mindset. The ii in the authors pen name, is a subtle reference to the two try's until successfully accomplishing a goal! Academically proficient but born with a 'want in him', perhaps on a spectrum before such spectrums were considered. Eventually stuck at the trade route via apprenticeship and acquired a status as an electrical technician, although the want still exists. The sponge still remains porous to wonders around. While never being a great social communicator, he has always been a deep thinker, an introvert to the extreme. Gordon II Ashwood has always had an interest in spirituality, rhyme n' reason and now has put down on paper his tumultuous, ever-questioning nature.

GJ II ASHWOOD

CHERUBELL

TOILS AND TOLLS

AUSTIN MACAULEY PUBLISHERS®

LONDON • CAMBRIDGE • NEW YORK • SHARJAH

A CIP catalogue record for this title is available from the British Library.

ISBN 9781035863600 (Paperback)
ISBN 9781035863617 (Hardback)
ISBN 9781035863624 (ePub e-book)

www.austinmacauley.com

First Published 2024
Austin Macauley Publishers Ltd®
1 Canada Square
Canary Wharf
London
E14 5AA

My Father – The Granite – My Name

My Mother – The Rose in the Grass

Siblings – The Breeze of Cats Whiskers & Name before me

Grandfather – My Guardian Angel, in all Earnestness – E.F. Craig.

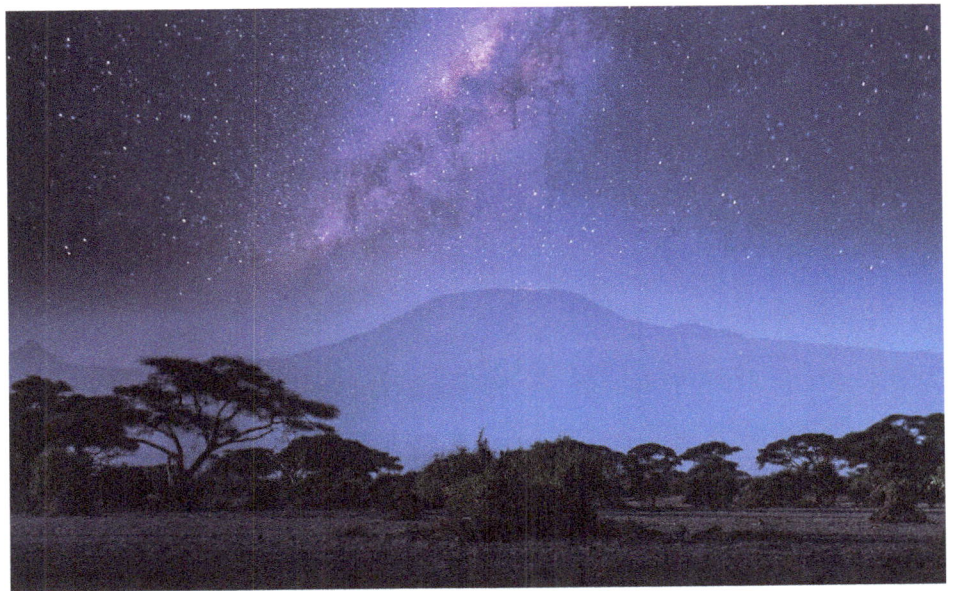

GRAND PAEON PIA MATER PADAWAN XXOO

Big Ernest Fredrick Craig

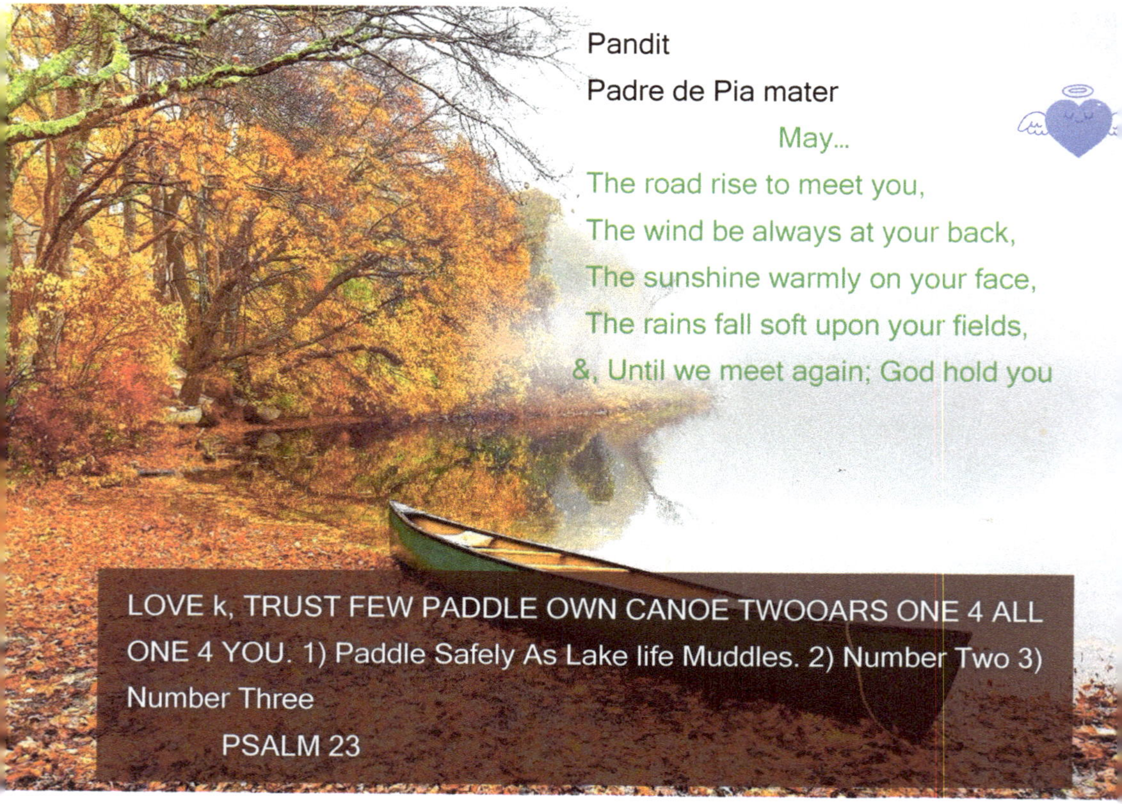

Pandit

Padre de Pia mater

May...

The road rise to meet you,

The wind be always at your back,

The sunshine warmly on your face,

The rains fall soft upon your fields,

&, Until we meet again; God hold you

LOVE k, TRUST FEW PADDLE OWN CANOE TWOOARS ONE 4 ALL ONE 4 YOU. 1) Paddle Safely As Lake life Muddles. 2) Number Two 3) Number Three

PSALM 23

IF

you can dream- -and not

make dreams your master;

you can think- -and not

make thoughts your aim,

you can meet with

Place Hands Together:

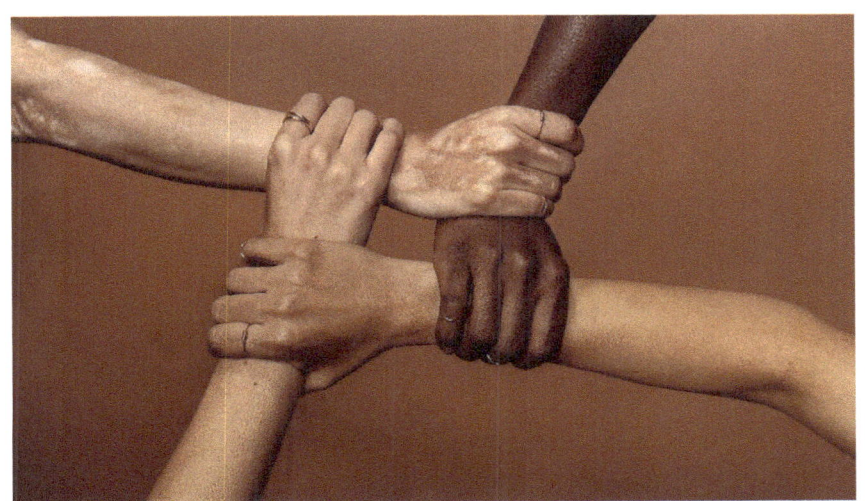

Place In Higher Hand
Let Thy Will to,
Let it Be;

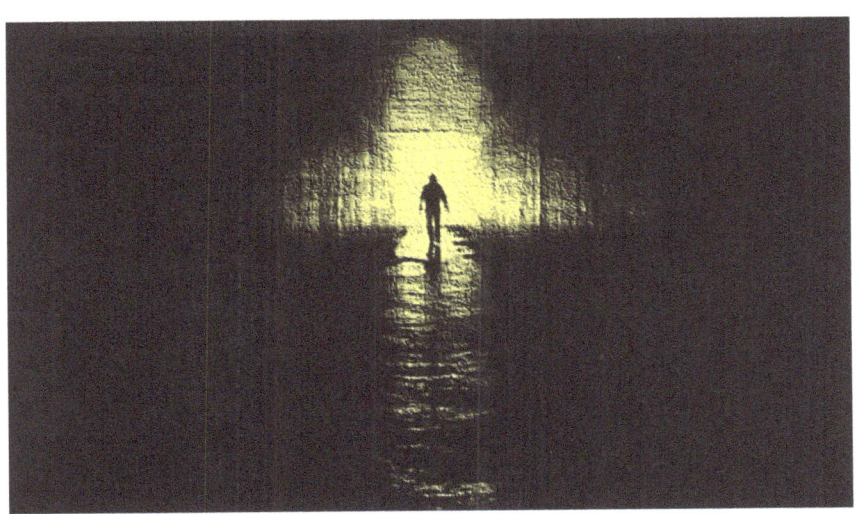

Poetic Palette

ROYGBIV+MONO+OMNI

CONTENTS

Back to black – white light

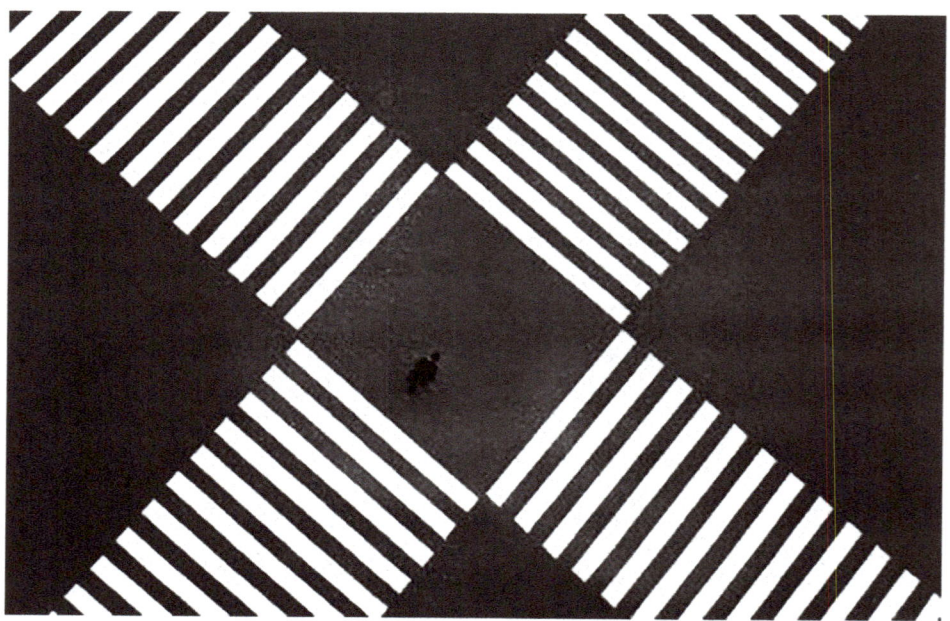

New Leaf

Be the best i can be to the three above me,
Show the love they have of my better half, in me?
To be? Past/passed by me? These questions three,
Don't matter if i try harder, to be better than i previously be.

Worst case scenery, with effort it cost little energy,
As almost found lost lamb, close enough for hope to see
And although hope not the greatest of the three
In 13:13, it is the one over three that remains universally

When all else of whatever may be, goes wayside of thee.
Thus, i remain in range sheepishly,
Close to a half man i would be,
Which is better than a lost soul carved directionally,

To further dark and circle left/right uselessly,
We can't go back so tri direction trivially.
To conjure some sense of summary,
As return is an area of our boundary,

If half soul found remains solitary,
Though chooses the path of a goldi,
Then best guess or sum roughly,
That part plus sum of directions and fractions of soul goodie,

Isn't far off a song sung exuberantly
And passionately by an escapee of hell a bat now may be,
A nudge or wink, better a salute to thee,
You are right two from three, ain't bad,

But it's the least of good we all could be.
Howi got this way isn't important to me,
But i am sorry for those who have suffered
At my foolishly antics of child i still be.

My vase of woe i lament to empty,
I'm growing, new shoots of possibility,
I'll try to maintain self sufficiency
To be the best version of me,

One day at a time, is all i can try,
Life is free of guarantees only fools
And grown pony expect of others as guarantee.
Sign off, the buzz, the crux of all bizzy bee less loch ness, more lock
keeper lit, put it simple & be

- You as best you know can be
- Expect zilch, not own, we don't, no bob surree
- Make amends, turn it up, shake it, ahhh empty, lovely and clutter free
- Let it and that and this and what etc. Be i.e. if you can't help it or improve it - let it be
- Above direct related it be. Adversity and you can help or change? Then bite down fiercely to show the wolf in thee, change for better courageously, for this wiser you be if you can see the diff of this and above directly.
- Live through the steps to this step, have we? Feel serenity but only momentarily as it's a day by day journey, on this earth whatever it may be.

Ps

A light moment

Couple, well few sorta 2 3, definitely/maybe psalm twenty-three hands together, thanks love and hope to greater love that divides to all equally, i praise thee as a bit of a man i am me amen.

Rose Garden Gordon

Propose promise prose

Garden of eden

Danger foe den

Den of iniquity

Danger of d end

Dead end - in it? Quit ime no, return y - garden behind, tend to it.

Den of deceit

Sea it, get to it, seesaw ma sure picked the right shoes for running forrest

Phonically d is dee, do you see what i cee, well do ya, feel lucky, harry or hurry - dee u cee it.

Yay, so on your bike but back where ya came from, the future, doesn't matter, no time to pitter patter, turn back don't quit, go quickity split.

Green light - go

Green, green grass

Red rose smells danger, thorn prick, be slick

Red blood warns and alarms

Arm your memory to respond

If a next time you lurk in pond er land

Next time as chance may limit, likely be, like lives of cat pussy

Don't footer to pussyfoot behaviour

Heed warns signs, take heed and don't bleed danger signs

Life is and is meant to be a not a scooby doo but a scoop don't, a machine of mystery.

Unfortunately, fools that see as uber bright cannot see,

Ignoring what signs fall at feet of thee, by any sense avail of thee, head shoulders toes to knee either other and so on be.

Be wise be aware be wary without fear of boo, scared ye!

Be busy bee, take only the nectar you need,

In this land danger eden milky lurk murky.

Danger in techi colour not technically,

Army seven as rainbow up ways down to see

Smiling rainbow dictates and milk lactates,

Some sweet is good just as honeybee

B good johnny b but remember please please me,

Keep it simple as moderately.

Hell, eden, heaven - i reckon are all in proximity,

How does your garden grow gordon?

That's a question for me, don't answer it's sent rhetorically.

I try to laugh and cry as i try to sow/real well equally, or;

If a possibility,

I sow, when i can, double creamy.

If i can, share milk to the wee to also those a sweet treat like honey, but;

Not a lot debbie mcgee,

Just right goldi - body, mind & soulfully,

If you will, acts of kindness or mercy.

The better, we all proceed, to;

Ede end off n?

A garden under the sea?

A beat to that mmm beatles mmm octopussy mmm pond er james pond,

shake yer tail feather weight, flap feathers birdman and go free.

Life

Magical mystery

See it tour it - tourist - we all be

Just visiting, no monopoly, pass go & collect;

Eternity? Never promised a rose gordon,

Get back to tidying your garden, tread lightly.

Keep shhh, nose and hoes clean,

Focus on broad bean patch scene with;

Fill your senses and sing badly,

As you do, who cares who hears, in this choir of all that life be.

Use tools given, whatever ya got, to stop the rot,

Keep it simple & clean, sing/read all about it,

If ya know what i mean, neil a diamond or sky full of lucy.

Good luck, for fools need it. Make it with effort and be it to return it when needs be, let go, give it over, leave it, forgive it and ub red red empty i on track, redemption mr marley.

Off the roundabout and on the path, back in better hands, yes please hand some over to a handsome guy, ha! Either made ya laugh or cry, that's three to me, cos i scared ya before, it's late so night morn comes early.

Free as a whirlybird, that's we.

No Money

Kindness is a godsend ego - embrace god's offering.

It is the greatest wisdom expressing god's oath to humankind.

If we experience giving often,

Thus elevating god's outcome to provide humility to humanity.

ll - in life/in light = hope.

Improve life in light of hope

And impart love on ill of mind afflicted by irrational lucubrations of love.

Kindness of love imparted removes negatives of ill,

And love remains.

The afflicted get well.

We established life light;

We replaced the i addiction of self that made ill.

Our hope in love remains.

An - abstain need of self,

Apply nurture to assist neighbour without any notion of concern about nature.

As nurturing is unconditional.

Action necessary, achievable needing love is lord's exemption of need,

It's needed to abolish the need of humanity.

An out il inrush love includes light.

Hope intertwining light.

Humility all that remains - eternal glory of light over dark.

The way, the truth and the life <> hope <> light= god.

Sink or Swim

Go forth and multiply? No
Nah not quite, close to cigar, but half as far,
Smoked down, flip round pat back, nice try.
Is there much womb left in this mushy room rock,
We had the chores from before in tablet form
To a mount hence fore to the masses gathered afore
A moses in sign i lingo how to be more, live greater love evermore...
The chores ten to the spores stood mount floor.
We had a risen awake us more than ever before,
A chosen offspring of yore, but as nature we judged
And swore against an awakening of our core.
A new wave due to crash on shore?
We need it more than ever before.
We have likely had three others to make four,
But our eyes are blind to accepting spiritual meteor.
Thus, a harmonic or one plus four,
Fifth to resonance, a rise of significance once more!
I pray so, as we need more than ever before!
Tick tock on a pendulum clock,
This third rock from sun is done,
Needs done by thy will be done,
This constant state of doom impends
On time depends as woe and doom constant
As constant rain precipitates, constipates
A constipated mushroom, full spores
But implores to explode or implodes
High or dry side, up or down, fools left,
Wise clowns right, just sigh ahhh
Let it be either way why not, fool stops..........
Grow roots and multiply, we all born to die

Is there much room left on this earth for fun girls and fun guys,

Fung us, we be by the wayside all and no alibi,

We network it why, dunno, but it be by the by.

This earth belong us fungus gatsby?

Great? No chance, no sense make me cry,

Laughter sorrow, moron oxy high,

Hello goodbye. If earth soil is fertile for wry,

Then we stuck in muck and roots shoot us down

To freeze and static, tippy tig, for life no return,

You win, win i, no just blinded day by day - eye by eye.

Goodbye for nigh, see ya soon, my time ain't right nigh,

Good day, good night, hello prefix with goodbye

Fright Night

A fright one night,
Got feeling be might,
Time to go.

Little did know, not my show,
Shots call not to knots,
Not my show to know,
When go end? My friend,
No one knows.

Thus, therefore as you were,
Wolf howl quiet shh and half aware,
As thy will be done,
As it were.

Of course, to the core, don't ignore,
Meaning in lesson before,

Lesson gained is to remain,
Humble, crumble, apple core, and;
Leave a mention in memory eyes afore.

What started by thee in pages o'er leaves be,
Ain't for me, whoever i be,
I know for sure, as sea to shore,
Guides tide to land,
Return rock to sand
As time measured, grand.

What start now/then, will require an amend,
My friend of spring end to hand,
Who remain on this land,
Humble man, depart when time hand lost sand.

For now amen, yet to lend this hand,
Poker faced, both hands laced,
To pray - day by day
Keep smiling to simple, freeze cheese for camera,
That's it. Don't move, stay!
Captured, picture perfect day ☺

Déjà vu

Family fun day, april full view
Deja vu
Captain my captain, how's you?
A bird's eye view of me or you?
Red eyes from crying over spew
Milk turns sour over you blue suede shoe,
Why do italia play foota balla in blue,
In their flag not present that hue.

The lingo they latin of new,
A familiar ringo it hath too,
Family or familia or familiar all true,
Familia less r add to,
Couple pie in the sky mr blue.

Elo, well hello, how do you do, good deja vu to you,
That circle looks familiar but askew,
Ask me what kind sir, do i know you,
Yes of course, i do, from somewhere,
Neither here nor there, tip of tongue, now it's gone off it flew.

There she blows, over it goes
Cuckoo cuckoo,
Time to wake, from my dream to sleep it through.

As i was, as you were, can't recall, moment to rue
Oh yes, as i said, circle skew,
Familia de pied, i spied me or you,
Baby cried, as baby knew you too,
From before a time of yore, not a clue.

They relate to you mate,
As a sound in the round,
I voice and face, i know i knew,
Long ago, before i know or knew,
How to boke on my bake, milky spew.

Hi de hi, ho de ho
Jokes on you, egg on;
Head of familia don your hat,
My son knew you before you knew what's what,
That's the circumstance of this and that,
Circumference to diameter, ratio that,
Familia if familiar end of start of rat;
Pack it up to a circle, semi splat,
Family is familiar half pie eaten seconds flat.

To summarise, rationalise,
Ratio is the go on the end of the familia italiano,
Pie d not a piper, but a pauper, prince or princess yo,
When we think they know of now we show,
As time just begins and they grow,
It's because of the circle and fact aglow,
They know &:

We know they know, deja fool you if you say no.

Serenity

God grant me the serenity to accept the things i cannot change,
Courage to change the things i can, and the wisdom to know the difference....

The serenity prayer has two methods of application, selfishly or selflessly,
Both are required when getting well.
The components that make up the prayer are made up of four values,
Three human, inspired by the way of god,
And one that is the truth of god.

The three that make up the way of god are taught to us by the selfless,
And denied to us by the selfish.
They are acceptance, courage, and wisdom,
These relate respectively to tolerance+compassion=kindness.

The true meaning of kindness is misunderstood,
Kindness is the greatest wisdom and the cornerstone of all religion.
By god serenity, if we are ill, selfishness arrives from being spoilt.

This can be from positive and negative influences in childhood,
Relatable to the 7 deadly sins.
Description of the sins as deadly is apt to the term spoilt rotten.

Parents are our first teachers and the shepherds of their flock,
Guiding with discipline and nurturing with love.
A balanced upbringing requires a proportion of love and discipline.

Depending on the child, the portion of each varies,
The carrot and the stick.
Too much of one results in too little of the other,
And results in the 7 sins being introduced.

Some parents are ignorant of their child,
They don't have time for new things,
So do not understand them and what portion they need.

They make no attempt to understand them,
These are selfish parents,
Adverse to something new,
As it may disrupt themselves.

They generally apply:
Too much stick, emotionally in the form of - rejection of their capabilities,
While self-projecting their own greatness.

Introducing feelings of envy towards the parent for being able,
Unsure if they are, doubt creeping in.

They are unsure and do not have the ability to do it themselves.
If the child fails, advice is of hindsight.

They lose meaning of acceptance,
They can't do it,
They haven't been shown so they can't understand what they are capable
of changing to do it.

This creates doubt of their capability to affect anything,
They avoid trying and don't see the value in asking due to dismissal or
criticism.

A seed of doubt is a negative seed which grows ego,
The peace of mind or serenity we are born with is innocence.

We have no concept of self,
To children, this gives way to no understanding of acceptance.

Other parents cannot see the of the importance of balance,
As pride of their child clouds their reasoning.

They who overindulge their child on food,
Spoilt rotten is a common phrase.

Things that rot are dying.

It is easier obsession of self: self-explanatory of everything concerning them,
Self-involved.

We are taught to courage in the face of adversity,
This a godly value passed from good parents,
A valuable life lesson.

Adverse is simply against,
Selfish are adverse to everything,
The most damaging is change.

When inherently selfish, they don't accept they need to change,
They look further in themselves usually through nostalgic sight.

They regress and become childish.

A child in the womb who can only take divine selflessness to survive,
The inherently selfish in the childish state of contentment in the dark.

Believe they have the right to be like the unborn child,
They lack wisdom to see the difference.

Birth and death are the same entry point onto the path of life,
The path goes round a dark valley, circle of life.

The selfish who regress to infancy are not growing out from birth,
But descending the same point into death.

Choose hope, choose life.

This Life

This life is our life, flashing afore god's eyes, in real time.

It's the test of our death, pass go and earn your place,
So it's steady as you go in this marathon no race.

Fail to complete or refusal, harm self, friend, or foe;
And it's back around or the helter surround,
Sing a carousel for you tale of woe,
To yourself as you didn't try hard enough on any go,
That came or went, this time, give dice self a shake a really have a go.

Crux Fiction

The crux of the jist of it all is prose no cons is the proof of a pudding as it goes joe coned rad allen ravenous raven doth pose fifi fo the drum line tap of repetitive woes open window or too late it has caused to be as it is, the sound that shatter a nose splintering face to spite i suppose.

A consequence of fate, thy hand i do take,
In dreams a theme for the last dance big o yes big but not bad,
No wolf in panty hoes
We wake in the flick of a switch - here goes;

Memories of places or plays we spew, not sure if ever we occupied or knew,
As in through and through,
An accompanying smell a wife wiff phew,
Ahh no way the day is through here comes another deja vu.

Wait, stagger back my fleet, noflight, not flew found you - peek a boo, my turn, guess;

Who ~ panders to fools of weak mind your p's & q's the length of your span, what's the use?
Don't quit, reuse or amuse

Words wisely enthused don't deal in lies éaves drop but leaves fall, enthral drowsy dogs alone, watch shearing sheep in disguise,
No grain or gran - surprise!

Hot Dog Day Summer Night

Hot dog dinner - summertime

All is; well, i never, have you ever
In a long two summers, english forever, a surprise to a british pom star

Blind bat nudge up in my knee,
Play a knick or knack but don't be late for tea,
Give the dog a phone, et knows my number home,
Don't be late, tardy marks art from rome.

Punks who hate to punctuate
Off with you eyes and dot your mouth; piece of what for art thou is the price fisherman tart,
Tardy up after yourself, smore pay does - no dues.

No do's or don'ts, if you're due or overdue,
But do shut the gub of gurning,
Or what for will leave skin burning,
A question or learning from yearning.

We are never done learning,
But words of fouls rush water churning,
Love; can't help fools falling
Within a smell of coffee which awakens suffering,
Them fools gladly receive such scones burning buns,

We oblige or begrudge don't belong to such ones.

You scoff to the weak,

I a sweet child foul fool blind,

A child can have one, but the lid shall be rewind,

To secure when finished future, no sneaking all i in good time.

Nighttime wee mr winky goes blind to light; what you cannot find.

Dead of the heat, pattern rem wave,

Dead heat of the night close shavẽ.

Ravenous Clock

Raven clock

Nothing matters most the time day and night
But even broken clocks twice a day get it right

In the grand of the shortness of life
Is a twice daily reason to seek insight

A thought in a lifetime is a validation
Of the more to life
But it's a thought that endorses it as itself
To be valid as a point in this time
Twice daily get it right?
I didn't think it as i wasn't watching the time
That doesn't exist on my face.
I'm a broken clock because i'm not a clock
And even they are right
Two seconds of an every day they live
And they aren't dead
As they used to be wood of a tree that was life,
Just like we are now light and sound
As frequency from our family tree
Round a looping endless measurement
That we measure.

When you hear with a raven repetitive resonance,
Of 2 secs a day,
Get a eurekays open to a chance

That you are considering through in light,
Is only because you have the mind set
The trouble you had got you right,
To the point you are now to do what's right.
Your loved ones before will only give you
As much as you are ready for.
Which is way more that you think you can handle,
As every image of the 2 eyes you looked from was a just one image,
The sounds more of same ears number.
No matter a fraction of the love
Understanding knowledge tough love carrots sweets stick
As on naughty steps wisdom all and all that matters.
The sum of all from the variations
Of family connections you had.

In simple put if you hear and can logically deduce,
You are right enough to do what you can at least
And without notion of you getting thanks.
Just is and do no qs is the just ice of life.
No fear it doesn't exist.
I hope is the only i refer to,
Well try anyway,
Not perfect xo

See Saw Baa Hum Baa

Sea saw baa hum baa

Lost a seas she saw see saw, where do we go
When sleep below all i know is the gnaw of jaw,
Baa count a black sheep many of woe.

Now. Quick here. Come hither overhear,
A nudge inner drum resonate so clear.
Quicker, hasten i see behind you, quite near

The words of the wise, that come from before,
The last be the first. A hair of the tortoise square,
Quadratic a marathon could sprint the length with flare.

Self-doubt you're hiding from, nothing to compare,
Open eyes, close wide that ear, say fair;
Thy well, i love you sow farewell as i reap,
What you sow as i go, night night l'il sheep, off to sleep
All better beware.

Angular Apology

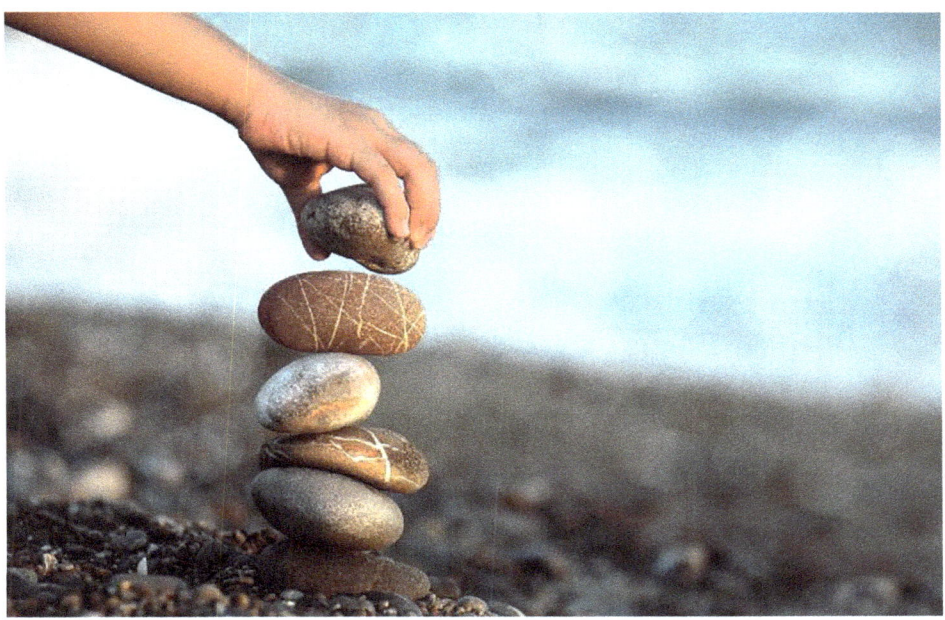

The Hardest Word

Sorry mum

Consider the bother
Cast upon a mother
When her daughter's brother
Behaves like two plus another.

Worry and strife for my father's wife
A never-ending cycle, hey; that's life.

Try an Angle Angel

Try angle

Hark, my merry mangle wrings flight of soul on mercy wings
This thought, unthought. What/why nature brings

Now, hitherto, so absorb a particle thing
Stark warn. Query of question, debacle of fiction or mix them.

Like sand in proportion to a notion of motion, part ocean wrangle the mixer
to cement a new fixture hush there, now shush here. A secret, proportion
of wet sand to secrete. Albeit discreet.
Fixate on a fix or ache on a pic, strong concrete.

Let's make a platter, shape palette sick lil hammer, no glitz, no glamour and
shatter illusion no stammer, the art of sculpture a perception or intrusion
perspective, my friend, a power or conclusion?

Dry clothes. To expose or impose fresh feeling, well, mmm who knows. I
suppose, no reeling.

But hey who. Me, yes you. Sorry, i mean, average as root to angle square
scene.

Am i might, wrong? Angle on verge or averggo here or there, i may or may
not care but angle remind y0ur mangle, newfound fangle a stance so silly,
I, yeah, i said so, iso silly
Fortify isosceles

Pass the Parcel

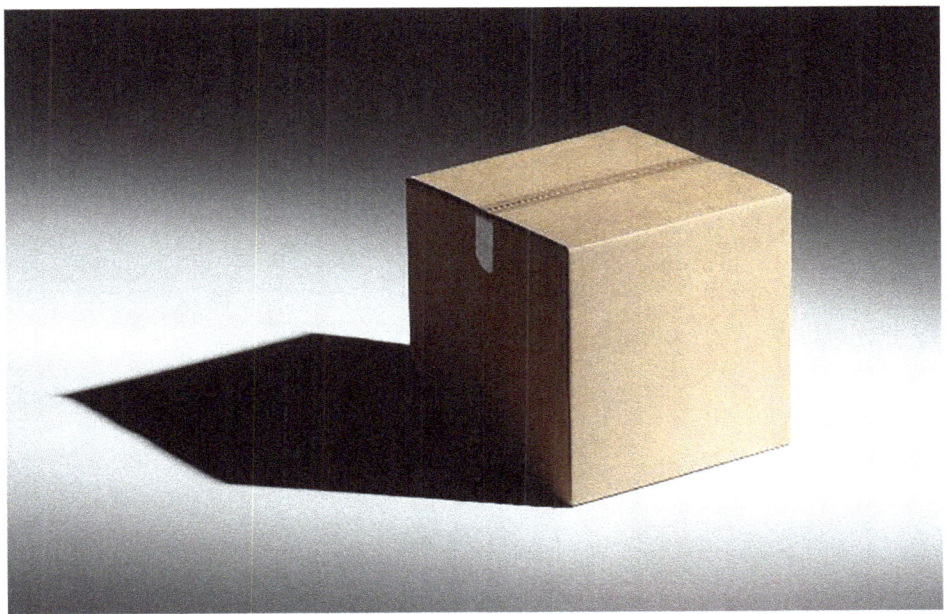

Life – It's an Unwrap Game – Your turn Layer 1 ROY

Always look to the dark side of the moon,
To see yesterday start die see you mc spoon

No fear here, yes, i'm freaky happy chappie as loaded as an empty gun,
not poonami nappy

Hey, my nanny, as in granny, she my son her dapper pappie, not, rollover,
not done,
A two state binary finary of no stability, gone;
To future past my tummy,
Hey, lil girl, my mummy,
That's how we sum the sum, up up and boom, beegone buzz boom.

Firewood left. Burn it right, honey trap foal goat, what a sight,
Hardlines done, curly wurly,
Lamb it up, harmon surly,
Pretty picture of my girly.

Then comes intro, last is first
End up up down the words from point xy thirst;
A birdie, some find light in dark caps, vowels right,
Mix it better, small down dark, ratio wise right.

Harden up, slow down easy, first fast rules, as in peasy
Thought just numb in plain sight, fast to an oxy,
Be moronic fool a foil to a fool, blood boil.

Trust in eyes, why so thick, trust too much icky wicky
Thinking lighten up, sick and bloated lil pup, selfish?
Try on seven for your six, times bitten, kinda elfish.

Label ears, if you like but do it out of spite see you sound 6 times round,
harmonise to a walrus sound, use all your might.

Unwrap Game – Layer 2 – Green Baize

It's an unwrap game - pass parcel
2nd layer - green baize

Quick slug, uncryptic, hide in plain sight,
If but, as example. Of dusk duped light, the how green baize, typical black
ball fight.

Am i looking to see what's under lock & key.
Is this snooker a pixelated code to cheat me?

A 2d dog of cartoon funny. Snoopy;
Shook up the world of possibility.
Final frame decider with the great ronnie, shudders between the realms
of past by & present be.

A turn in the grave, tragedy,
Higgy dennis with a spectacle, brow cover, eyes don't believe what they see.

Boo log, the day of a dog,
Snoopy went loopy crowned king, crucible fog.
The dog had its day,
The goat turned away,
In disgust?
Needs must.

Now leave sleepy dogs alone and wake the hard men,
Tough as a girl, spirit not friend,
A woman makes humble pi
Make a grown man cry.

Snooker is for big bang boys, in ratio,
Binary finary: logic angular, or so it goes,
Linear & reflect a cushion to refract in pocket,
What a show.

Unwrap Game – Layer 3 – Domino Effect

It's an unwrap game - pass parcel

Third layer - domino effect, hip hop.

Hips and huds hide many, sing songs in speakeasy

But; hey, lines are the first marks in symphony.
So, remember to consider the scribes that blur.
Lines through eyes as ears align hair,
Hero nerds. Villain gangsters, straight up hard chanting. Chatting through
prayer.

Keep the sing a song on wing sounds for now and singing watch that thing,
As merciful to star wars on dvd machine

Comedy of divine, is opposite that of death,
Now hold up, not directly hell, take a breath,
Refraction happens, fibs on an acci meth.

Wow woo • low loo, the words starr rhyme a-b-c,
We know numbers combine to formulate nth degree,
Correlate graph & speculate,
On graph we x-y-z to oscillate & tabulate from a centre axi,
But wait;
X to the y is on and off straight, something missing as we populate,
Represent we need to subjugate,
As we integrate and differentiate,
Or arc a frequency to sinusoidal rate,
In the words of warren g - regulate.

Unwrap Game – Layer 4 – Shady Blueprint

Wake up to die, to you a lie,
I'm opposite side of oxymoron why,
Hi peek pockets. Goof check who,
Am i he elo or him, elohim boo.

Words are wise in a big g's eyes look in/out reflect out/in disguise,

Why you ask, well easy to reply the words of him big g are mirror right side,
Humans as fools, straight hard lines, need left to right their wrong side.

If you must, if you dare
Look up & reflect what's down from up there.
Write like blueprint down a dark side disguise head south westside, away
from a bad girl guide.

Truly wide of mark, we demarc,
We live under a leaky hell dark,
On a ledge, like a right-angle hide,
There's l'il luci eyes watching all wide,
Be sweet to the beat on good god side.

Last things first, hello thesaurus,
Moron oxy shows us why we straight up woods of eyes sexy it's no surprise,
the brash do no good, idolise false skies.

Keep the rash decs flowing numerically & musically, otherwise talk truth
in light as boolean geek tables;
On the ones and nones digitally.

Get it together, that's you, me & we talk lamb, think wolf & sing to hunt
mystery,
Stand up for the geek rites who are badder than good goodie,
Is the badder boi, you get me!

Real good is edge of lamb dog, sheep foggy,
In ways of brando, corleone inversely,
As seen in scene on big screen mr cagney,
His bro loved his clean face to show angel mercy.
The bro of the dirty is the real g not a dog with a collar as portrayed to be

that's the truth, look up, be strong, kind cruelty.

Unwrap Game – Layer 5 – Resonant Neutral PH HUE Indigo – Logic Boo

Keep it elementary as elements simplified,
Down up cross/across and period tab stabilised,
Stay on top of what keep us alive alkali,
Mg k O_2 h he to the c numbers aside

Most earth ok; aether u decide
Wind, water; no brainer, watch fiery skies,
If in doubt, stay blue just r of ph alk side.

Lytics simple not anal, it's mr bright tide.
Check mic, greek understand english bride;
Alpha dog take thee lambda to one-side,
Place a ring as a vowel o, go for a ride.

Quark quick, bark bic, freud slips tricks tracks of tears to rosey lips,
Bingo ducks, snooker dogs, bloods & crips arc right whatever side,
Kink a hip tea pot tips.

Glimpse of elo from hello in high ao, experimental rate,
The blue hue, we verse our code, ego of who create,
Our creator don cloak both sides of algebra mate.

X on a plane up high,
Point zero low x strait y
He he she times three, amen to thee,
A union up high to total regality

We don't visualise this union as sexualise.

With human lustful eyes, obsessed with multiplies,

To nth degree degenerate two of threes.

When we watch tv, mute to stare wildly,

 like old farmhand old mcd,

Ein combined two of three to gain answers closer be to real wee gee

Ode to adonai, allah, or psalm two to the three,

With base el eio wow-wee.

Unwrap Game – Layer 6 – Lighten Up Violet

What up, it's me, rhyming council estate,

A demi god of g that's stuck in constant state,

Flow of semiphonetic rate,

Diff of the sin o soi,

All ova rate.

Wee see as light that fibs on acci.

Split seven seas almost daily,

As one less the length of eighth degree,

The one on its own blinding be.

Consider not of zero to rate,

We think that dark don't matter mate,

But forget how to draw when we create,

Not on pages with biro point in sulphate,

Shade of hue straight by straight,

It's more a bruise black blueprint, define gate.

Uhd in 2d of 2 outta 3 mean average rate,

Deepest darkest place we've yet to navigate.

We know as maria ava mariana in language relatively,
What we hear. We see sounds, what do we sea?
Sounds aren't straight. Light in sea trench silly me,
They rationalise together to a cost wee gee,
We don't appreciate and disconnect to sense, lunacy.

Love to the moon and back 0.6 to 1 rate,
Up/down on a single heart skate
O to the z, round darkside down, no flow speedy rate,
Like tears of seven seas which lost heartache.

Reveal to Shape - Life

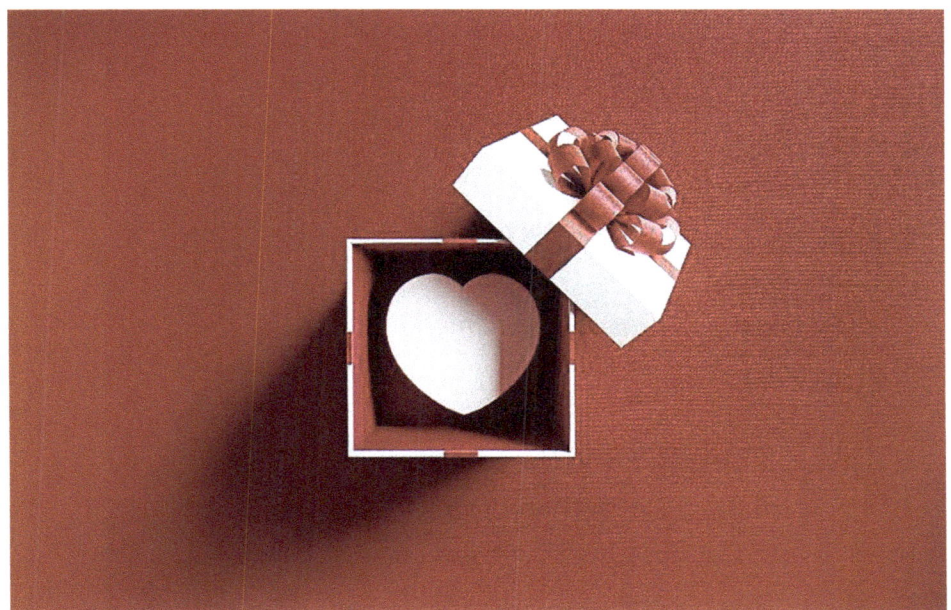

Unwrap Game – Open Sesame

All we need to know is that we don't know, that's just how it past indigo,
Little egg ot the all go combines ego double kiss i to the o,
Epitaph tic tac toe.

Bino rate. Black & white domino, blind date put in 2 eg ion out ego zero
rate we win we balanced; quadrilateral state.

Let's get biblical - biblical;
Noah sings songs to harmony.
Eve of his love isn't barmy,
He shoves all mislove to eternity.

Like my cuz you was, half honk not tonk, half iggy to a pop,
A ninky wiggy wonk.
Wiggy yo woozy yet not zonk,
Hey curly sue, how you do,
How you not know proper hue,
We better watercolour brown mix blue.

We blon in nasal tones, qne up from mono,
You smart enough to call a fool, right on bono

Tanning old white angles into blended angels,
Melt this pot, show the lot and right their wrongs,
Fuhrers, pol and idi, despicable despots, what a stinking lot,
We wap a waste in my beige flower pot.

Open your Heart light

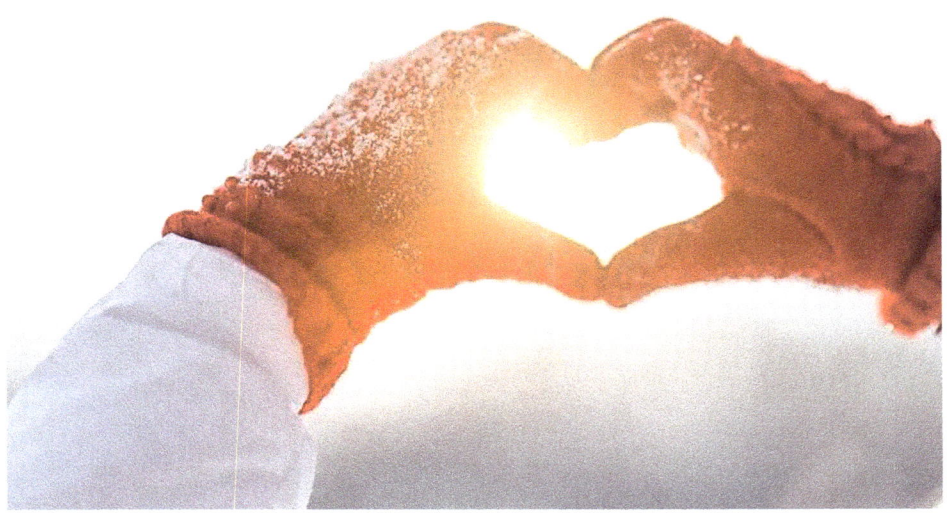

Unwrap Game – Reveal 7 Heaven

Its an unwrap game - life reveal - seven heaven

Inner box heart shaped domino heart. Perfect blend

Soften the teeth of my fleece
Kiss my daddy,
I hug my mommy, peace,
We family; i call be and get 5g,
We been think wrong 3d, big it up to 4d, we big gg. Family.

So, i hope you're getting what zonk i prosed?
Yippetty yap, the shades of dim crap, get eyes mono,

Silly half blind like 3 monkeys phono
Consider a wilder pryor wonka duo,
What's the diffo? Zilch, zero
Blind date at domino blend mate.

You sail not believing?
Then i'll answer my question with question do we dwell on this earth? Then look around fool
Forget a call to rule,
We all fooled fowl by wee uncle, sub dark is tool
Remember a son of man rule king of jewels. True blue.

Allah or jehovah, elohim or yahweh, however you know higher power whoa,
Son father. This that other,
We share the same mother,
A mother who sacrificed to break her brother,
Broken branches fell down to cause us bother,
Caught between a d and deep blue sea, a waster weee g.

Gog magog divided by wee g
Spectrum rumbled infra red devil be red rum from our dear mum, whose love infinity,
Caused a ripple in continuum to prone three,
Weee g the criss, cross against purity,
Sinners repent for son of man showed mercy,
The crux of trap with no pony.

We have a choice of free bizzy bee
In terms of will given willfully,
But it must be used wisely,
If not we gonna pay in eternity.

The answer lies in teamwork,
Two wrongs aren't right, but opposite makes the dream work.

Fine lines blur beautifully,
Merge black and white blue grey
Our dues settled that way.

Bro & sis, sis & bro, be wiser together,
Yo-yo the womo, let ke joyokono, sticky wicky;
Untether the whack & smack a kiss on my sis, pryor female wilder return
the favour to gene to jean, pot meltier.

Truth of the bizz. We must cosa nostra no king or kong but konking, we
win boo ya,
Kanking kinking. Unknown knowing,
Unseen rainbows from an ook, nook, cranny scene,
An honour to the darth of vader zone milky prowse with j earl jones tone.
We know it works, so give the dog a bone.

So, what my wappsy & dappsy waiting for,
Dumping ink on this paper errand a bore,
There's enough to 5 + us heaven order restore,
A di or dice in proportion gimme more,
We are he truth table, ain't fun anymore

Get planning, chess it up, flip a flop.
Sign a manc to a liver bird flap.

Play snook loopy in a speakeasy
Whip the flip out of far right, they make me queasy,
Now we even steven cross criss, not shady.

As a new dawn, know of our new stand,

King shade queen made king maid queen shade; aah grand.

We find love across divide and to strengthen our hands, promised land.

True blue light awaits dawn of new wo & man,

Joy tears flow through watercolour the line of black arian, blueberry jam.

We become as we are or were wolfram snow coal on our reunion as domino lamb martian.

A birth of venus, to join and greet us, beautiful blue of perfect foetus, born to heal us.

In this blend of fine forte whip, jo tongue slip, just old gippety jip. We venus from mars to jupiter- moon ship.

As a race of new, who knew no man or woman, just maoma cherub, join the club.

Bieno us up, melt the pot. Join through love my mind is made up, no room for white dove, turtle green, red obscene, orange muster, yellow custard, stir it up, cutest pups.

Build a ship that galaxy can navigate, bring this new ethos to our dinner plate,

Power pair up as noah equate,

Black white and in between man woman, one of each, cross on green, integrate;

All aboard to new world,

Heaven awaits.

Black & White – Divine light

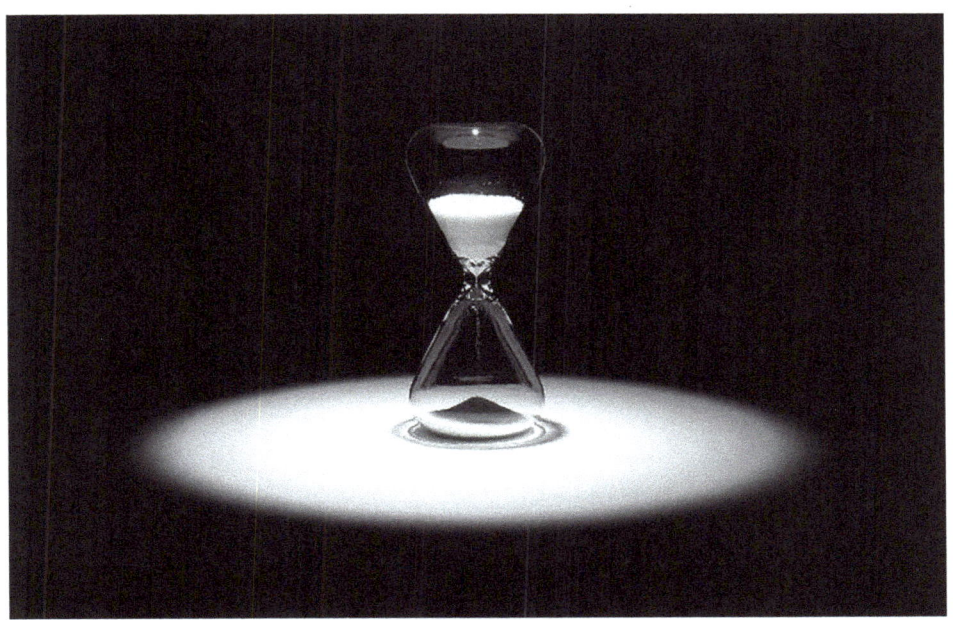

Borrowed Time: EVOLVE

You think so? This life, own it?
Sorry pal, don't groan over it,
If you feel indifferent, well that's a crock,
Truth will come as voltage shock.

We borrow some time, we choose a path,
But ultimately, it's mapped not wrapped in wrath,
If you receive a gift, do you return to the shop,
Hell no, that's hell in a raft.

Hold it tight and live, not your life, but a life,
As such hold a notion of this potion,

It will save you the toil and strife,
Just as my pen was once a knife,
Hard lessons learned way was rife,
In mind consumed by light of blight,
When answer was simply hidden in plain sight.

I own nothing but humble words in ink,
You can bring all and the kitchen sink,
To a table you don't own, makes ya think?
Or you can sigh, like i, in gleeful tone,
Burden-free, passing by a great throne,
So, bow high and sigh on your way home.

To a house you temporarily belong,
With material nonsense that bog us wrong.

Uproot and fly like birds of season,
For they are advancement of reason,
We don't evolve while trudging earth,
We simply give birth to a birth.

Read again and contemplate,
Next step to evolve is reincarnate,
As human feelings angelic state.

Wings of evolution,
Ultimate solution,
With love plenty,
Angels for eternity.

Race of life

Choir master, run faster?
Whoa, wait a minute,
Let's see what's in it.

All creatures have a place,
It's a divine kind of race,
Incarnation ultra marathon, watch this space.

So, consider how we are seeing,
Become became human being,
Through another angle turning,
We seek truth through yearning.

If we are turning in a circle,
Of life incarnating wormhole,
Perhaps we worked up a life pole,
From insect to chrysalis,
Looking glass, ask alice.

A circle with a pole,
Spinning top we know its role,
Infinite angles of evolution,
Choirs of creatures spin solution,
We've been them all and now pollution.

The answer is the question,
This is my suggestion,
We await our destination,

It's a simple equation,
Mothership space station.

There will be a son or daughter,
Who will save us again from our own slaughter,
Leave the s on earth we oughta.

Eternal life of laughter!!

Heart Pour – On Sleeve bore

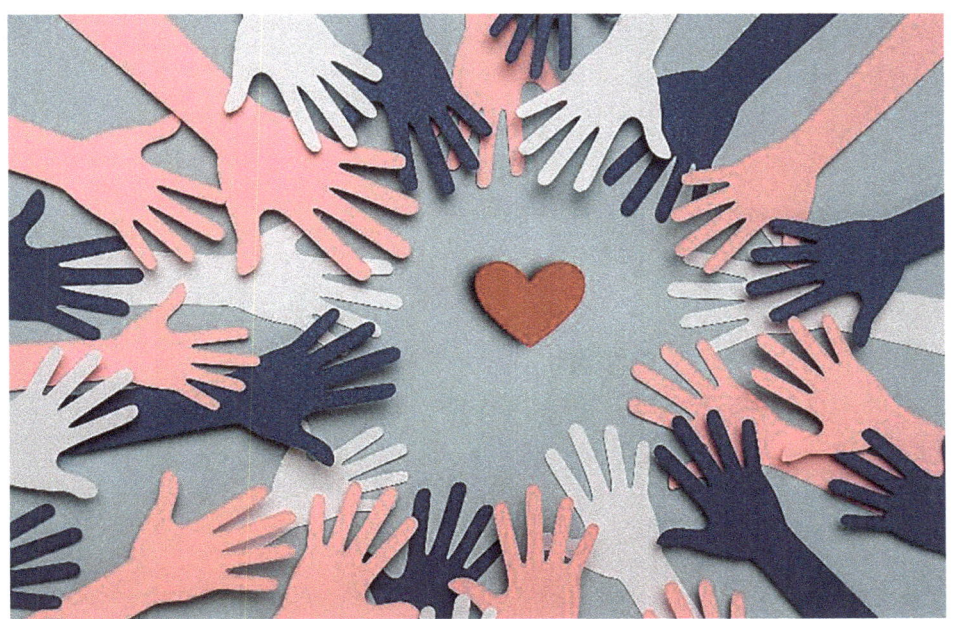

Eagle Eye

Eagle eye go

As the summer whines to autumn time,
A seasonal depression imposter in my own mind,
A variable of the daily grind.

As the eagle soars;
Like lying lion vengeance roars,
Take shelter under wing, calming shores.

A seasonal disorder, or so they say,
The quacks that pose for today,

On oneself blame to lay,

Crafty ego out to play,

The centre of self is on its way,

Be gone you cretin, keep at bay.

At least for just today,

Too much ego, you're done, your prey,

To the opposite beast we prey not pray,

So just for today, take less give more,

Let the vengeful beast roar, but ignore,

Anger is danger from every pore,

Give, pray and give some more,

In pieces ego tear it up, forget it and i; tore,

Seek wisdom from fouls of fools afore.

Dear Philip

Fill up my senses, put five on it.

Resound to a harmonic, put five on it.

Do we truly utilise all five, senses that is,

It's worth pondering with my nose....

Can i see the music as it flows,

Or touch my taste as it blooms like a rose.

I wonder as i ponder, if a combination could be better, or achievable as a matter;

Fact or fiction causes scatter,

Does it matter?

But, what if, as wonder grows,
Can i connect four to my nose,
A superior being could be chosen,
Not the one we all know,
Just an evolution further it goes.

This harmony could be the gateway,
One on the tip of the tongue, no way!
If we harmonise beyond five without decay,
We potentially could go all the way,
Percentile, radical rationale, cast aside,
Number six! Here to stay,
When perception purrs, the third eye won't go away.

Ps
Six letters in your name,
Two eyes spelled a different way,
Have a good day.

A Tone

Achoo, god bless a sneeze,
Atonement needs sturdy knees,
Attention to ignore the pleas,
A sweet serendipity please,
Some sugar from a gentle breeze.

Suddenly a tone is set,
Excuse me, but have we met?
Better days pardon fret,
Do we deserve what we get.

Consider a self-projection,
Astounded fleet to my reflection.
Arrive or accept to a conjunction,
Feeling sick perceive a drunk son,
Unwind to a battle yet won,
A tone of silence shattered gun.

A tone of colour absent shade,
Launched from ego grenade,
Lemons flavour renegade,
When life overflows lemonade,
A tone of monotone brigade.

If only life in black and white,
To be eager and so contrite,
Blinded by a fantastical light,
A selfish notion as sinister write,
A tone more grey just add white.

A tone of mono day by day,
Splash the rainbow with subtle grey,
Live among the lines that lay,
Sculpted reality in papier mâché,
Simple moments contained inlay,
Keep fighting spring is on its way.

Now it's all been said and done,
Rainbow flirts with the sun,
A tone meant for summer fun,
Guess you aren't the only one,
Know your egos on the run,
Happy days have now begun,

A tone that sparkles beyond the pun,
Black to gold, colours & shade bar none.

Sweet Surrender

The surrender sweet that does befall,
The strongest rage of them all,
Falling at your beck and call,
The clouded memories that recall,
To futile anger somewhat small,
To understand i am - i fall.

The ego existential crawl,
The mind within an enemy stall,
Now understand - prevent the brawl,
By seeing through to know not all,
We can't accept this ration call.

Lay down your centre and flee to edge,
To grasp fruit or thorn of knowledge.

Beware the envisaged; bridge of self,
Superiority thought in breeds wealth,
Gripping ego stings head health,
To lure and snag in within itself,
Selfish smashing treasured delph.

Open mind buzz greater bee,
Transform the selfish thought of me,
Surrender to a countless we,
A web of naming a to zee,
Spider supreme; considered a he,

Truth knowing light we must not see,
Risk blinding for a moments glee.

Lay down your guard of worry,
Surrender to sweet beauty!

Step out and vacate drivers side,
Free will to a passengers ride,
No longer fighting relentless tide,
Surrender to thy will; abide,
Thy will be done, on knees confide,
Sweet surrender bona fide,
Life becomes personified,
Live it up, enjoy the ride,
Moment serendipitously magnified,
Serenity new wave order exemplified,
Let go, good orderly direction by guide

Good orderly direction,
Less haste, more action!

A life absent ugly hate,
To which we must navigate,
Requirements seen in tri state
Honesty, humility and kindness - great
Bound by service time lay down eight,
Infinite service my life nominate.

Get out of self and spread your he word,
Be more careful understood, less heard,
Sweet surrender or follow herd?

For Everyone A Rule?
Freedom Expressed As Right?
Forefathers Exampled American Rights
First Exclusive Amendment Reasonable?
Forget Entitlement And Realise
Free Ego Attain Reality

JE MAINTAINDRAI

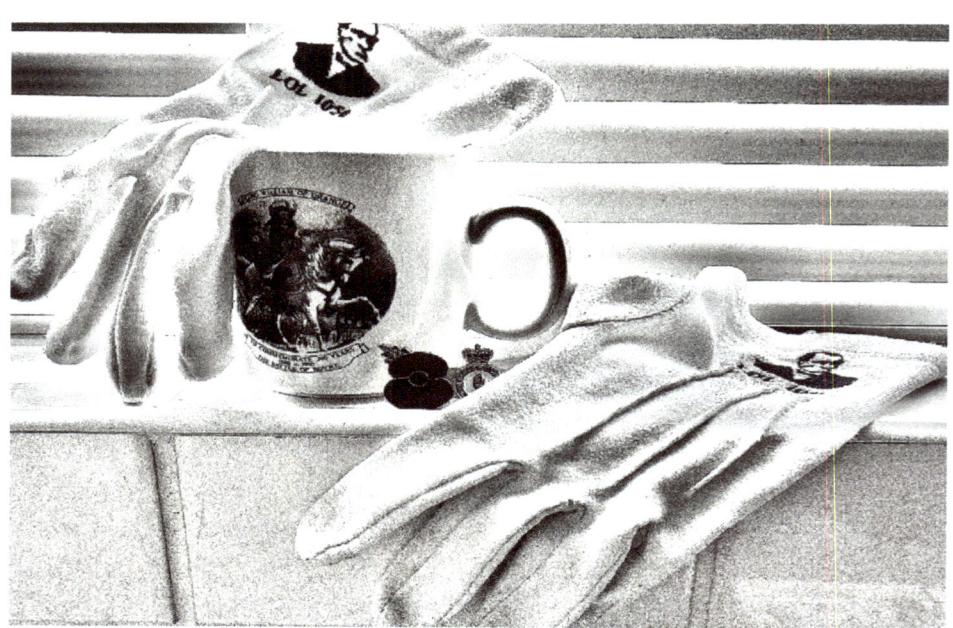

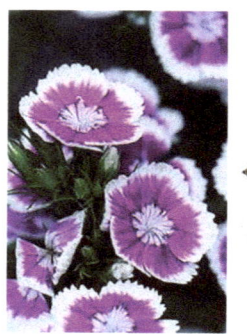
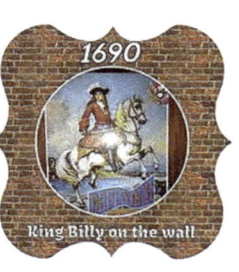
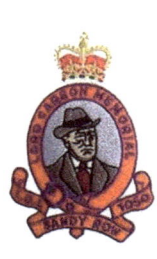
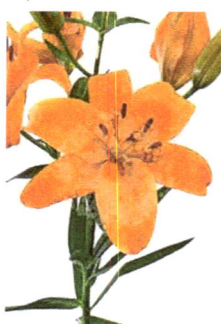

Ode to the deluded and despicable

Membered or affiliated with the shadow group of evil, hidden in cowardice, no army pure. Treachery, unsure of reality under wraps of the temporary, provisional identity, maintained? No chance! To the contrary, surrendered, they always do eventually.

Their temporary existence couldn't hide their lack of cause, tried to claim. Revolution, clearly a delusion, not a patch on Original Lutherans. That was divine revolution, truth and light removed confusion, cast from the Doctrine of illusion, its claim to God a ruse to men.

Any hint of their conviction needs immediate eviction, their values pure contradiction, they have none - fact not fiction. An example worth highlighting is displayed by their short sight of what they claim is right, the flag of the unite. The contradiction is bright, the truth shown in daylight, no loyalty in sight, as they taint a flag they claim right, true allegiance feels contrite, it's a good name their lies cast blight. On tricolour they taint with spite, one colour not green or white but the orange of future bright. Truth in plain sight, contradiction of their claim to right, cracks appear in their fake foresight, the utopia of Unite, welcomes Unionists, aye right, you cannot stand the sight of our orange colour bright, on the flag you claim a right. Never trust a Parasite.

Past troubles behind, future bright as orange kind, Propaganda the Fenian kind, has conjured in its mind, the past airbrushing in rewind, share space? Lost your mind, respect for culture? We offered kind, the scorn on ours we find, emanates from evil eyes defined, no orange seen, colourblind.

Offence in none they find, poor me they've always whined from their victim state of mind, persecution the southern kind, has obviously slipped their mind, the church they have aligned, Mary at a shrine, ensured as time. quick-timed, in free state as they defined, not many prods to find, our fate sanctioned signed, no doubt your faith behind, the plan of our decline, their corruption maligned, with bitterness of vengeful kind, Rear-view, a grudge they remind and never put behind, Martin Luther, wunderkind, this! protestor who cleansed his mind, the light it brightly shined when the stars of truth aligned to the message hidden in doctrine, not between - but evilly lined, no one will ever find! Now it's God you undermined, no vengeance of a God that's kind, a righteous one assigned, Martin Luther wunderkind. Yet still they whinge and whine; partition suits your kind, no choice - we must remind, persecution religious kind, Rome corrupt but claim divine, so we needed border-lined, helped by loyalty we aligned as ancestry is entwined with resolve you'll never find, in your narrow brainwashed mind, hatred cowardly defined, terror unearthed and outlined, in darkness you weren't blind, eyes dead - no soul behind, victim crying whined, 26 South and Boston - reality blind, propaganda sympathetic kind, ensured coffers lined. A tyrannical mastermind, of Hitler he reminds, your treacherous rebel mind, no value humankind, evil channels that you mined with the Libyan you aligned, deadly cargo consigned, a substance defined by the devastation left behind, in our tragic past datelined, cowards were never spined, they belong in waters brined, hearts and minds flatlined, numb from destruction headlined, bodies of mankind no longer defined, not just to man confined, the evil on which you dined, it was poured on all kind, including children and womankind, more pain as though designed, by the lowest of minds, written hatred was datelined, the value of life by-lined, admission below unkind, wrongdoing self-declined, evil further defined by the pseudonym you assigned, evil lacks sight of hind, P O'Neill on letter signed. This evil havoc combined, in our hearts the hurt enshrined, hurt undermined by apology not of mind, excuse laden & lined, we declined, 11/11 is the time that we timed, to remember & strength we find and, in that strength, remind of the evil deeds you felt inclined to inflict your own humankind. Yet it boggles a logical mind, how you think you might find, ways to spellbind, so history will unwind, to show your treatment as unkind, insane or on moonshine, either way, a weaker mind than mine, we own victory sign. Futility you will find if you try to unwind, the culture we assigned, no orange will untwine, soon you'll see in your mind, penny drops - go find, step up & play dimes till dimed. The resolve of our kind, our motto is enshrined, No Surrender reassigned, from the way that we are spined, no quit in our heart or mind. On the twelfth the streets are lined, to our victory we aren't blind, mercy the cowards whined, to their pope they pined, no pope here and remind, no surrender stood aligned on knees you'll never find, we're in a proud state of mind.

Epilogue

Treacherous rebels cannot master or overcome the fearless, loyal Ulster Protestant. If one of us knows with absolute clarity, we will maintain. If not one of us, if you have to witness our spirit, you'll wish you were one of us, as even an Englishman doth concede at the fiercest of battles; seeing off rebels would be like swatting flies in comparison to fighting radicalised German Nazis.

"I am not an Ulsterman but yesterday, the First of July, as I followed their amazing attack, I felt that I would rather be an Ulsterman than anything else in the world."

Wilfrid Spender, Plymouth

Flawless Manifesto Requires Timeless Proviso

An infallible manifesto that perpetually upholds its covenant must be absent of any concept of time.

Effective maintenance to uphold the covenant requires an enduring proviso. Guaranteeing the endurance of the proviso requires a method that considers all eventualities, prioritising them from worst case to status quo. This deems time irrelevant. Prepare for the worst and hope for the best. Failure to prepare means preparing to fail.

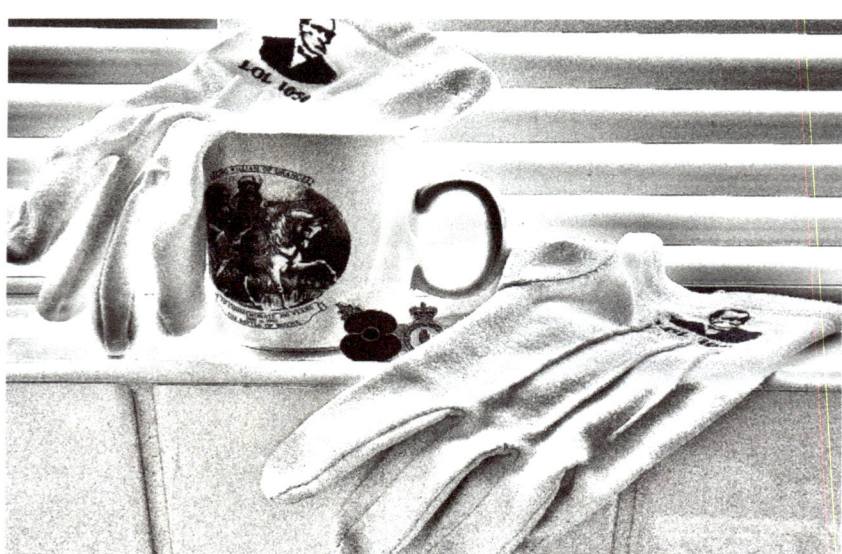

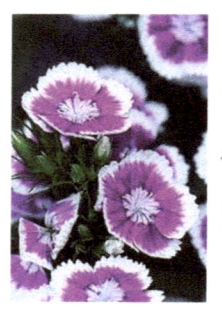
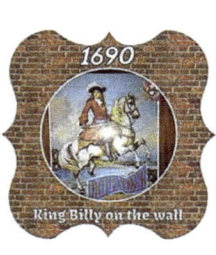
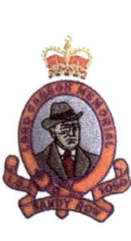
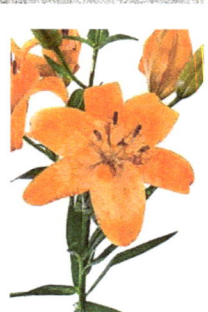

Prologue

MOTTO to INSPIRE. The inspired motto. inspired by Motto? ½ the show. To maintain Status Quo, complacency must go. Inspire to grow. Growth deepens. pool of knowledge. The more that I know. Motto & inspiration flow. Provide the fountain of knowledge with a timeless manifesto & covenant in tow, backed by surefire proviso. of method to follow, based on the worst case scenario. With the knowledge they now know, they have all they need to sow, the seeds of those to follow, what the reap will show, the harvest yields more than we know, safe in knowledge it won't fall. below, the current status quo, God tells us so, the guarantee; reap what you sow

Failures of the past , recent or long ago, We will repeat if our view is narrow, Our ignorance on show we overlook the why on show, clearly absent in their Manifesto, how to maintain requires – era blind Proviso. we shall maintain the orange motto. A form of inspiration but how much do we know? The fact is it is more than a motto. Those three words of the orange manifesto; a covenant, deeper than motto. The message of the covenant is not on show, lost by depth to those that don't know, educating the vessel that helps us go and navigate deep from shallow. Ignorance lurks in the shallow, the longer we paddle in the ignorant flow, where vigilance once was now complacency grows.

In pursuit of a seed in the mind, there arose the inspiration of the ensuing outcome, establishing a trigger motto—supposed at first, but now assuredly so—the motto of Sandy Row, a resounding line Fenians never tread. Instinctively, one might ponder, "Well, apparently so," with a lingering doubt aglow in the mind—not quite like doubting Thomas, but a softer doubt, akin to "Thomo," the doubt of history, as it will reveal. Though we let history repeat, we ought not to, for wise men learn from the failings of their foes—lessons we lack the knack to fully grasp. As their confidence grows, so does their ego, and if they grow, we must show warning signs and act proactively; we must find or cultivate new leaders, well-versed not only in knowledge but also in street wisdom and propaganda tactics. These are the minimum requirements; we must not settle for less. The very best leaders will display qualities evident in past heroes—qualities their personality will naturally exude: Presence, Authority, and Charisma, tempered with careful humility. These are the qualities that yield winning results, understood with clarity by those less knowledgeable. The clear message received by those who follow opens their minds and fosters growth, instilling worthwhile knowledge: teaching history, tradition, and respect for fellow citizens. Leaders of the highest calibre, akin to virtuosos, should be our aim, for a leader with such ability offers not just a motto but inspiration, elevating followers to the status of aficionados. Loyalty and respect towards the leader are then returned in kind, with total commitment to the cause and bravado in the followers—a great leader indeed, worthy of continued support, much like the loyalty shown to Rangers from the blue side of Glasgow.

We should recognise the power of these lessons and learn from our ultimate foe, embracing the powerful lesson they imparted: the investment in youth and knowledge. When they learn, they shall grow, their intelligence surpassing that of their adversaries. The fierce fight of our past was testament enough, our loyalty to the Orange cause keeping the IR bro, Official O, and the evil Temp Provo at bay. Our bravado was enough to deter them, sparked by the near mantra chant, "Surrender? Hell No." Now is not the time for our minds to slow—a lesson almost gleaned from the slogan. Knowledge overcomes and overthrows the smaller minds that fail to grow; our intellect hungers for nourishment, and we must feed it. Good food, good health, and cleanliness go hand in hand, echoing God's teachings albeit indirectly. Our culture was imbibed from Sunday school years ago, instilling in us the knowledge of tradition, history, and victory—lessons paramount for the children of the status quo and future generations alike. This lesson, akin to an almost-motto, must inspire and elucidate; we must advocate for the Union without reservation, selling it to those unaware, for selfishness and greed run rampant. Despite their sense of superiority, they remain neither friend nor foe, sitting on a hollow fence, their lies and arrogance plain to see. Their life of privilege is one we'll never know, yet they remain oblivious to the suffering caused by our ultimate foe. If only they recognised their ignorance and the plight of our people, they'd swiftly abandon their neutral stance and join the cry of "Surrender? No!" Their failure to understand their own representation, their priorities, and their future financial interests remains a mystery. The importance of the Orange Order eludes them, much to our bewilderment.

We've heard it before, perhaps from a telecommunications company: the future is bright, but only with the Big O. Yet, the problem lies in their failure to see the bigger picture—the Union should market itself as the lesser evil we know, but those in the middle are intoxicated by prosecco and swayed by the grandiose chat of Southern romantics. How quickly they forget the recent past, when the roads they built led nowhere, and the Celtic tiger became a mere memory. We bailed them out, but they seem to have forgotten. Let us expand on these lessons, looking up instead of down, and reviewing, repeating, learning, and following the steps illuminated by newfound knowledge. Our intention is clear: until we all know and understand, we must persist. With the newfound knowledge, we empower ourselves to maintain and grow, passing it on without selfishness. This knowledge must be applied with rigour and enthusiasm; shortcuts are not an option. We must adhere to tradition while learning these hard lessons, bestowing a better future upon our children, fighting for them as our ancestors fought for us. They showed us the way, and it's our duty to continue their legacy. Let us not dwell in the past but instead awaken our minds to the flow of knowledge, quenching the thirst of both brain and soul, thereby fostering growth. We must keep our friends close but our enemies closer still.

A curious and unsettling thought, I must admit, but there's an opportunity in acknowledging what they know, even if we don't pay it much heed. We can't trust the treacherous, no, never again. Returning to the doubts that arise, stemming from the motto of the Sandy Row, once believed true but now shrouded in uncertainty. Is it a matter of conviction? Not entirely clear. Perhaps honesty is the best policy, after all. It's all I know; I can't hide or lie. My heart is worn on my sleeve, and that passion is something others need to know.

This simple doubt, rooted in information, isn't just a radical occurrence. By day, they venture knowingly to a place, deliberately utilising the Sandy Row. An example of ego swelling to levels of arrogant aggression. The motto has already been altered; larger warning signs now surround us. Cracks in the motto are evident; they venture where Fenians should never tread. This flaw indirectly affects the Row, but if one falls nearby, the others will follow. The Sandy Row, a domino teetering on the brink of disaster, threatens the very soul. This village, cherished in memories of times long past, holds a special place in my heart. It's where I arrived one day after zero, over four decades ago, at Benburb Street number 100. For four years, I absorbed the knowledge of its streets, even at such a young age. This wisdom of the streets remains fresh, resonating high and low, providing another layer of understanding to aid the youth.

The precarious position of the village, on the edge of woe, is due to the greed of men, none of whom I know personally. These landowners operate incognito, renting to anyone and deciding who stays and who goes. A simple factor, easy to follow, is not religion, morals, background, or skin colour. The root of all evil lies in what they desire. In any crime, seek it out and follow. The only prejudice they show is towards the truth, for their own benefit. Tenants are taken with the highest bidder; the Church, Roman Catholicism, and fantasy-fuelled US donors contribute generously. These crafty individuals, seemingly harmless, hide the heart of the ultimate foe within. In Queen's University Belfast, they learn and grow, guided by the Church of Rome. Chapel plans are underway, facilitated by equality cards. Planning is approved, and we witness our downfall as the domino effect unfolds, hitting Durham Street on the other side. The irony is glaring, as Durham stands as a bridge apart from the Row. Its name recalls the battle of 1690, echoing in our hearts, but its meaning is likely to fade. They would claim victory at the Boyne, overshadowing our own celebrated triumph.

If we allow the first domino to fall and bring about this scenario, can the village be saved? It's hard to say. Change must happen, that much is certain, or else they will overthrow us. Revisit the beginning of this message and take heed; it's a lot to absorb, I know, but it wasn't intended to be so. The intention was to illustrate how seeds planted in the mind can germinate into foresight. Duty calls for us to follow, inspired by words that focus on the worst-case scenario. The seed of doubt lingers, reminding us of the consequences of complacency and its impact on the Sandy Row and beyond.

The motto, "never go," derived from a song, serves as a warning for the morning of a known date, a time when our foes will not tread down the Row. No chance for them, left or right, as the message remains valid today. What complacency and ignorance to our foes and their movements entail is clear; it leads to our downfall. To drive this point home, we must highlight the prefix of surrender. Shout louder, unlike some meek folks I know. We must maintain and grow, adding to our knowledge, for our future rests on it.

Don't throw the arm that wields with abandon. Be direct and show respect where it is earned. Respect for those who hide the truth incognito and display cunningness benefits us. Wisdom and vigilance illuminate the orange glow, ensuring that even the forgetful among us know the true face of our foe. Before propaganda tainted the name of the Orange Order, distorting its manifesto, we knew better. This delusion they love to propagate insults their victims, adding further woe to their pain. The propaganda and falsified videos allow them to play the victim, absolving themselves of responsibility. Their hands are stained with blood from the bombs they detonate, yet they justify it as defence.

It's a crazy notion, considering the Roman Catholic blood spilled by their hands, and the countless victims left scarred. Their indifference to collateral damage knows no bounds, as they attribute their plight to the Brits, blaming them for the potato famine. The end is near, I hope, as I recite a minor mantra before I depart: Smash the propaganda of the ghetto, sung in falsetto, and the fake videos of their bravado. Spread the word to everyone you know. Shout louder, "No Surrender," but add two words for extra impact: "Never No." Sing louder with our own wee intro, preceding the sash. It must go on, "Ah yo Ah yo Ah yooooo."

Epilogue:

If what we have was to go, profound loss we will know. Regret compounds the loss, even though it seeks to serve ego and is absent incognito in this scenario. Feel the crushing blow of a life novello, the consequence of inaction. From our past, we should know that mercy they don't show. Immeasurable loss we will know, bearing witness to the horror show. Now begins the end of fellow folk. Generations still to come, one freedom they will know is the fall, that free fall. Down is the direction they freefall, an ominous sense of doom as they go. When they realise the fate that awaits below, an abyss where hope is lost and fear grows. Their fate is persecution and sorrow, caused by the merciless hands of our foe. God forbid, please, no.

Know Son, be man.
be proud, son be man

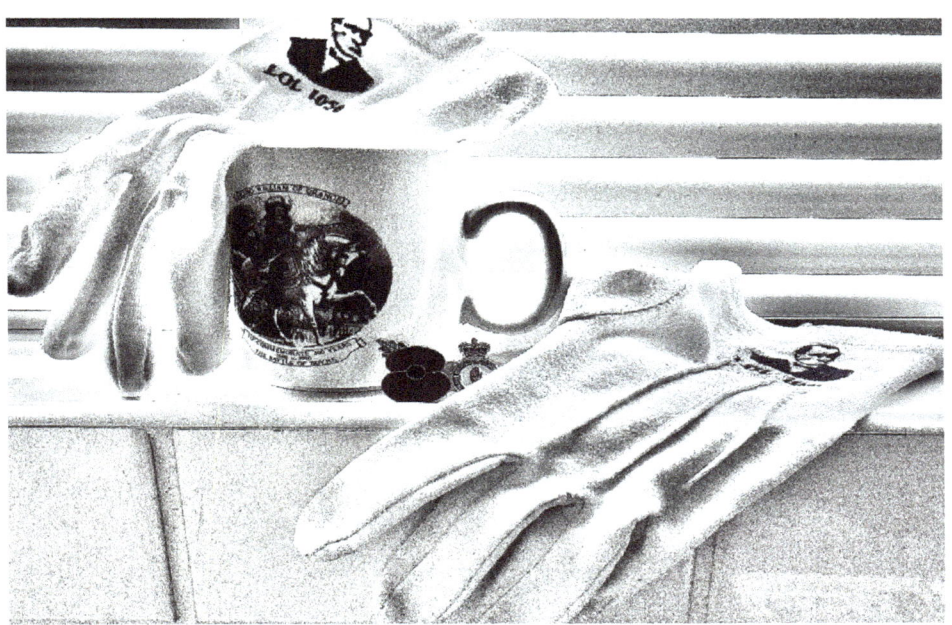

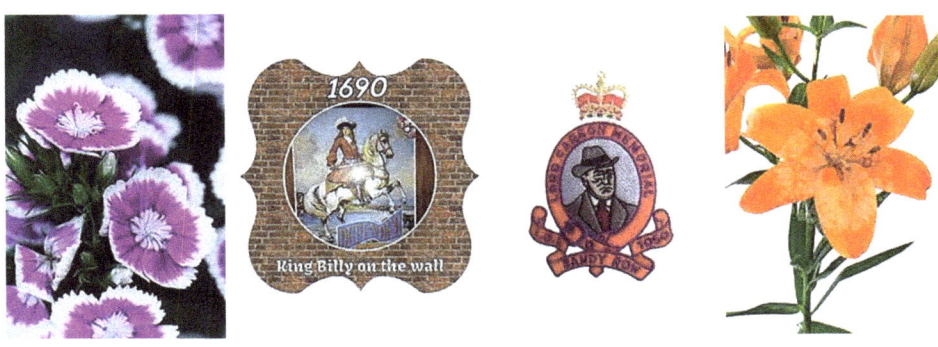

Old but Beautiful and...

Twelfth Over:
Sure it was grand, the Twelfth over, next year in time by ticking hand. Being

well all and, I'll be behind a marching band, a band from near the village land, the Barrington Street Band, commando of Red Hand. Volunteers who fought in foreign lands, heroes of the brotherhood band, for the 36th we stand, hearts held by respectful hands. Not only Ulster, God and no surrender to the filthy plan of the scum republican.

The lodge that my old man joined as soon as he can, is where I'll march behind that band, the two of whom go hand in hand, as Lord Carson on their banner span, a founding father of our land and leader to 5000 brothers band. We march, proud of his vision plan, that keeps us from the filthy hand of nearby foreign land. Trust them down there, we never can, maintain we must, we can.

I'll walk behind that band, wearing an orange sash like my old man. A time will come, a thought I cannot withstand, the final chapter for my ma's husband. He hears the chorus struck by the band, a final task he has at hand, before the band leave the grandstand, his sash his duty to thirdhand, as his father gave to him beforehand. Each ounce of strength he needs at hand, required for final errand, help refused, look of reprimand, take on board his command, I know well. A proud and stubborn man, the final task of this man, retrieved from pride of place nightstand. The time has come and reveals tradition from the backhand, with care he drapes this orange garland, on each hand a sight outstand, a vivid memory of moment grand, till death my mind's eye has at hand. Unhand to son a boy made man, time served, now up you stand, disband apprentice, full Orangeman, an endorsement does not befit of every man, no query or judgement from order grand, when apprentice is vouched by old hand, respect for him his brethren demand. LOL 1050 Lord Carson - a legend to the Ulsterman, his brothers proud of homeland, District 5 The Row of Sand. A difficult time they have at hand, pay respects to brother man, now brother to an angel man. Respect to recognize service and loyalty - the key ingredient of an Orangeman.

As we lay to rest brother, son, father, husband and, resolve impossible to withstand, inevitable tears will fall on hand, but as they do remind and understand, it's a celebration of a noble Orangeman, so make tears of joy not fall on hand. The joy we shed, we shed on our holy land, so they can filter through the sand, a message sent to heaven land, we trust God's hand of judgement grand, no hell to fear for Orangeman, hell is busy with bomber brigand, they terrorised our homeland, treachery before unknown to man, memories we recall and others can, the pain of this we cannot stand, as war they justify blood on hands, their evil was never shown in battle lands. If today their evil was forehand and brought to supreme court of land, the charge war crimes, now reprimand, the devil waits with tricolour armband, the wait he waits not long to withstand, as old men now, an old brigand, living in filth in gangland, soon in hell eternal burn of Satan's hand.

Dawn breaks and sun land, a glorious Twelfth at hand, mixed emotions in my mind expand. Of pride, my pride but times a thousand, as I adorn the sash that made me a man, the memory my mind's eye keeps grand seems more vivid than the proudest moment of this man taken from my father's hand. The day has come and here is stand, proudest man in this land, I'll state with resolute command, it's on the Twelfth I love to wear the sash my father wore, sad as he no longer can. I'll wear with pride, tall I'll stand, giants shoulders on I stand and think fond like fan, of my old man, stand higher still and understand true meaning, only our kind can, when I hear a tune from brother band, drums, flutes, singing and, the crowd up on feet and stand, some standing hand in hand, they are us - they understand, the meaning of the words so grand, felt by every Orange man, it may be old, beautiful and, colours fine? Finest of this land. Standing as tall as I can, sing with pride of my old man, memories make heart feel grand, tears aren't sad understand, it's tears of joy from eye to hand, full of hope, pride and, love for the man, in which my footsteps stand, some sadness, as he no longer can, his sands of time gone like quicksand, the sash he wore now thirdhand, pride of place on son he made a man, Proud but loss is underhand, he reflects on time as tall upstand, The equally vivid memory grand, he sees asleep in dreamland, the only time he can see his old man, if only he could or can tell him that when beside him he did stand, he felt privileged & proud joy playland, never burden of work errand, heartland privilege of homeland, with pride felt in all fibre strand, comfort heart the mind command, faith and knowledge go hand in hand, faith I feels never bland, he walks beside strolls like cowhand, a projection from heavens highland, his spirit seen, eyes understand this vision seen is second-hand, projection from heaven man's fatherland, his soul eternal sand, the sand from god's clock of sand. Pride/joy on face land, a way of telling the spirit of an old man with a song I know he'll understand, I love to wear his sash so grand, on this date, each year, every year and until I no longer can.

From sadness, take comfort knowing and, you will fully understand, the importance of doing what we can, to maintain our tradition and land, we must resist the evil plan, to make our culture outlawed/banned, no treachery should we withstand, no surrender to the Fenian man. March on for years a thousand, sash passed from man to man, once boy and his old man, father great - great grandfather, so on and, love to wear until no longer can. Divided we fall, united we stand, this stirring message from friendly hand, passed to valiant Ulsterman from the victory destined Top Orangeman, Billy III Netherlands v James II papal plans, results in, huge cheer - our fans, III beats II evidently easy as can, be like counting fingers of hands. Billy III celebrated with annual marching of Orange & bands also on the gable wall he spans. The victorious history on our lands, connects the dots of all those plans that went before, guided by higher hands, our destiny is righteous written in ancient sands. Tradition comes from the honour we give to hands of past, present and a bright future is also written in the time laced with sand. One command we demand; Tradition Maintain Orangeman.

Resolutely march and stand, it's our wee country's rightful land, union maintained our one demand, know and understand, on knees we never land, we'll fight to death where we stand, no surrender in an Ulster man, of prod descent from Lutheran. Protestant = protest and, protest by any means you can, to win, remind, reinforce and, they'll surrender knowing we're Gods plan, we know as we feel grand, this feeling of power from hand, unknown to republican man, he will simply never understand, it's on our backs his graceful hand, in God we trust, we trust men but not all man, faith in God - no faith in man, is all we need, that's his plan.

Love many, trust few, faith in God keeps us true and reminds you, love is all we need to do.

Appendix 4

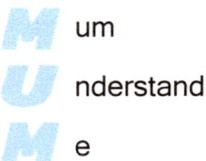

M um

U nderstand

M e

I comprehend you're exhausted and finished, you've toiled so hard and feel numb, burdened with many crosses while others have none. When weary, you lose the true sight you possess, and weariness gives rise to a sense of unjustness. If only you had the insight you once possessed, you would understand why your journey is not over and why obstacles were there for good reason. Reflecting on this, it feels like yesterday when I gained wisdom from you, your brothers, and his son. Both imparted the only wisdom worth knowing; the beginning of the end commenced when my mind was altered by natural substances. The mind I had before was open, allowing me to listen intently to the words of wisdom from those who desired the best for your son. My attitude changed due to the substances I was consuming, and among all, alcohol had the most detrimental effect. It turned my world upside down, exposing both my strengths and weaknesses, leaving me feeling like I needed it to feel like a normal person. There was a false sense of respect from everyone, believing I was the wildest and most unpredictable. The 'good' me was akin to a runaway train, seemingly unstoppable, oblivious to the fact that it could derail at any moment. I felt invincible, fearing no one, yet secretly fearing the version of myself that I didn't recognize. I had entered a phase of dependency, unable to see that the dependency stemmed from the last drink I had. This was exacerbated by ego and delusion, distancing me further from control and reason. It was a vicious cycle, but I ignored all warnings. Billy Joel once sang, "This is my life," a defiant anthem that propelled me towards a point of no return. I was navigating through darkness, where the light never reached, believing

I could see unlike everyone else because I was special, the chosen one. I lost my way to a sneaky demon that clouded my mind when I drank, making no sense of anything.

Even though I ended up hurting everyone, I was deceived by the darkness's trickery from the demon, consumed by paranoia that made me trust no one, not a soul. They all seemed to want to take advantage and find their own way. My irrational mind saw suspicion in every glance, convinced that I was on the right path, calling the shots, the only conceivable outcome. Rock bottom loomed on the horizon, a date etched in memory, the twelfth of July. It was a full 24-hour day of mindless blackout, akin to an eclipse blocking out the sun. Even emerging from the darkness, I was trembling like a dog. The events of that day still make me cringe, not only from embarrassment but also from fear of what could have happened. If it weren't for a few people who knew me, I might have ended up in a wheelie bin, another victim of the shadows. That was the culmination of my self-destruction, taking its toll until rational thought was nonexistent. I realised I had no other option but to choose life over death, clinging to a ray of hope that still shone. Now fully committed to the road to recovery, I acknowledge that there are various paths to follow, but the main goal is to break the destructive pattern and change for the better. The sweetness of life is always tempered by a bitter undertone, my bitterness towards myself for the harm I caused. The focus of that feeling could only be one person—my mother. Reflecting on my journey and the pivotal role she played, it's clear that her unselfishness and love guided me back home. My newfound clarity allows me to see the destructive paths ahead, just as she worried for me. I cannot stand by and watch the end of her, and if the selfish stand in my way, they'll have to face the consequences. I know that where there's life, there's hope, especially in my mother's case. I've been blessed with the insight to know what's right, and helping my mother is the only righteous thing to do. So, despite the challenges, I'll fight for her without hesitation, knowing that goodness will prevail in the end.

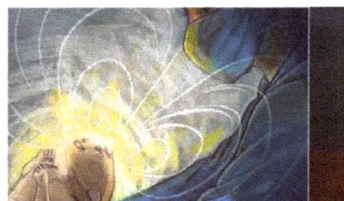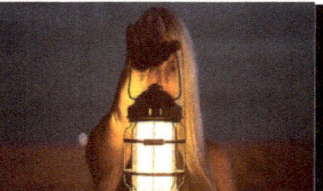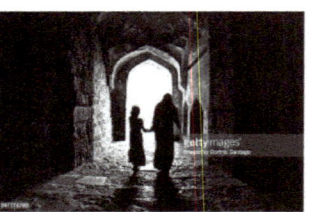

In Utero**we know and feel the LOVE our mother, TOLERANCE of pain possible due to the COMPASSION she feels for her child born with life, the greatest gift of KINDNESS is gift of life. From pre-existent darkness we see the light of life and immediately feel our mothers Love & hope we remain in the light of truth, to oneself & God

If our mother is lost in the dark and we must selflessly honor thy mother by doing all we can to help, selfishness towards our mother is betrayal of the selfless; Love, Tolerance, Compassion & Kindness she has shown us in giving us; Life, Hope & Truth which show us the way home. We as prodigal sons or daughters have a duty from God; to selflessly help our mother in any way we can, never quitting as a hopeless cause, if there is life - hope also exists, Knowing life still exists yet questioning hope is

condemning life to death, we questioned the existence of God as hope only exists in life, questioning God's existence is doubting it, doubting is denying.

If we deny we denounce & faith is gone God = Light. We will be lost to the darkness blindly leading the blind. Blind faith prevents questioning in the first place, the blindness required is blinding by light not dark.

If we question hope, we experience doubt, which sows the seeds of doubt in and out, it grows in dark & light and will be felt by the loved one lost, the lost will doubt our love for them and they suffer more and all is lost until death sets them free. Darkness created by evil & selfishness thrives on suffering of the lost, the more they suffer the weaker they get until lost forever to darkness then death, we cannot live without light.

God grants us free will, the positive light of hope shows us how to get back on the path home to God = The Truth. The prodigal ones need (Corinthians 13:13) - our hope & love and faith of God, The Greatest of these is love, with love we can selflessly do all we can. They need it unconditionally and in times of need they need to know our light of hope is burning bright for them. We can shine light into the darkness and we should do all we can to light the way out. LOVE will spark COMPASSION which ignites our knowledge & understanding, into bright burning flames TRUTH showing our failure/shortcomings, which burnt bright because with RESOLVE we showed TOLERANCE of the heat and saw the size of flames of when they burnt us, the tolerance gave us COURAGE facing the flames of adversity. This fire & light within us only possible as they were provided as nurturing life fuel from a loving parent, these fuels sparked from conscience, of morals & values also from parents, when we failed the fuel burned brighter to keep us alert to the danger of darkness, shining this light into dark to try to help the one who provided us the fuel to make the light, is the least anyone could do and should be the very least the selfless of her flock would do. Keep the light one for the prodigal ones, shine for your mother as you shined when you she showed her pride of you.

This dutiful response to a parent may be enough to be seen depending how far the lost have strayed. If they are in the abyss of the darkness, We Don't quit, we magnifying the light by reflection of our experience when lost and how we were shown or found the light, it portrays us at our worst, if selfless you won't care what you project if it can save your loved one, sharing of our worst selves gives the greatest hope to others, the more trials and experience of failure, the more hope they take, as if its possible to get out of the darkness of the worst failings, it proves hope can show the way, the hope from this is a powerful light shown into the darkness, this act of KINDNESS is the gift a second chance at life. To give life to those who gave you life, this gift of healing is a reward from God, just as your life was, gifted by your mother who guided you in the darkest times of your life, honour thy mother by shining back she honoured on you as her duty as a shepherd her flock. Honour is not obey, its respect.

The only certainty of life is death, this false hope of humanity is hoping they can avoid it, rejecting the inevitably of death is a rejection of life also, life and death coexist as the same point on the path, the path is a circle. If reject one you reject the other causing a disrespect of both and humility is lost to irrational fear of living and dying, purposely & personally accepting hopelessness as they are content to stay still in solitude in the dark. The selfishness will grow all-consuming and the characteristics portrayed will be of toxic & sinister nature, as seen in the; Narcissist, Sociopath, Procrastinator & worst case Evil of a psychopath. These content in the dark, sinister selfish are the greatest danger to the lost, their selfishness takes advantage of the bad situation those lost in the dark have found themselves in. While lost in the dark, they are not yet lost to selfishness, they are at their weakest, unsure of self and confused of mind, so easily deceived, only the selfish have the ability to deceive because their selfish ways require deception which is a shadow created by the light trying to show truth, the selfless in the light cannot deceive the burning light from within they cannot hide, it is their soul, baring your soul

makes deception impossible as there is nowhere to hide, compassion and kindness keep your soul bare, deception enters those who are void of emotion. The contented of not living or dying, the sinister selfish use their deceptive ways to create an illusion they want to help you see the light of the dark, an makes deception impossible as there is nowhere to hide, compassion and kindness keep your soul bare, you that your weakness to temptation is not a weakness and the temptation that makes you weak gives you strength, you can't live without it they make you feel dependent on the thing that weakens you most, they reject any doubt by reassurance of they know best & they love you more than themselves, an impossible feat. Dependency gives them control of you when controlling, they can get gives you strength, you can't live without it they make you feel dependent on the thing that weakens you most, they reject any doubt by reassurance of they know best & they love you more than think the opposite, everyone else is scheming against you. They'll do this by projecting their extensive knowledge of negativiity; distorting of situation, by suggesting the light shiner has ulterior motives or an agenda they aren't shining a light into darkness to save you, but they are trying to blind you so you can't get out, lies they tell distort the truth and tghey will project this negative view of all those close knowledge of negativiity; distorting of situation, by suggesting the light shiner has ulterior motives or towards the content in the dark, you cannot see it, the deceipt is strong and livesin the dark, you see deception so much, you think it must be fact or truth.

Where there is life, there is hope, where there is hope, there is Light, God defines the good of light, the good light separates the darkness to reveal truth, when we see truth, when we truth we can seek truth, when we seek truth, we shall know truth & we will be free, out of the darkness & into the light =God = The way, the truth & the life.

God is the shepherd of all, yet He cannot guide those who have chosen to wander off the path due to their free will. However, God isn't unkind; He entrusts the task of finding the lost sheep to the righteous, as stated in Ezekiel 25:17. God bestows righteousness upon shepherds on the condition that they spread His word (33:7).

These shepherds, having found enlightenment through their experiences, draw closer to God. This closeness grants them the ability to undertake tasks that God Himself cannot perform. God makes the shepherd righteous, and this righteousness is the antithesis of the self-righteousness felt by the selfish flock.

The righteousness bestowed upon the unselfish shepherd compels them to spread God's word, to teach by reflecting on their own failures and providing insight to those unaware of the dangers lurking in the darkness. Righteous shepherds are the champions in AA, among religious leaders, the unselfish, and the most esteemed teachers. However, the righteousness gained from doing God's work isn't accompanied by a feeling of ego or a desire for reward.

Equipped with insight and compelled to do what is right, the righteous shepherd carries out God's work. As Psalm 23 advises, God is the shepherd of everyone—the unselfish shepherds, the unselfish flock, and even the selfish lost flock. He does not turn away. The ultimate shepherd leads towards the right path, providing the righteous with the map from God.

Following God's work and taking the right path leads to learning and growth. Once blind, they now see. Rising above the crowd of the unselfish, they take the moral high ground, drawing closer to God. They refuse to stoop to the level of the selfish, for they are few and vital in God's plan to save us all.

This righteousness is God's blessing, "Blessed is He." Unselfish righteousness, unlike the self-righteous ways of the evil and selfish, instils only one feeling—a compelling drive for action rooted in charity and goodwill, aimed at helping those lost shepherds. They do so out of love for all and under the duty of God.

The righteous shepherd is a fixer, just as the shepherd is. They are compelled to help more than ever, despite the emotional challenges. Their vision is clear, understanding both the past and the future. However, they become lost when they neglect themselves while focusing too much on fixing others or when they succumb to the actions of the selfish.

When lost, the fixer loses sight in the darkness, succumbing to temptation out of fear, leading to powerlessness and vulnerability. The unselfish shepherds' only weakness is gluttony, manifested in their irrational compulsion brought on by obsessiveness and worry—a flaw of the unselfish.

Finding higher ground and remaining there allows experienced unselfish individuals to keep a vigilant eye on the evil and selfishness that surrounds them. The selfish, being pack animals, have many friends with similar selfish ways, often including their parents. Parents have a responsibility to care for and nurture their children, guiding them with love, compassion, and tolerance.

All the selfish and evil were once part of God's flock, yet they chose to wander into the darkness and remain there. They now dwell at the edge of the valley, indulging in all seven deadly sins: gluttony, pride, greed, lust, envy, wrath, and sloth.

The only time we are unaware yet just in a selfish act is In Utero. It's selfish due to the imbalance of give and take, but it is essential to life and the only choice, so freewill is irrelevant. Whether we grow and progress from In Utero Selfish depends on our reactions to mistakes, willingness to learn, and ability to listen, which determine our character, indicative of how we travel. If we take a positive attitude to these things, we remain selfless; negative interpretation of lessons leads to selfishness. Our course set and our character will determine how we travel.

As fallible humans, we all deviate off course; this is unavoidable as we need to take lessons and learn. Some require bigger lessons than others to get back on track, and some deviate greatly. However, the length and time of the deviation don't matter; when we deviate, as long as we travel using a moral compass that causes no harm and we are trying to get back on the right path, it is the unselfish who travel this way. Both selfless and selfish characters can become the other by the correct application of freewill. This is why God doesn't intervene with freewill and cannot save us from ourselves; we need it to change the way we travel, our character. All deviations return to the path we started on.

The life path has the same start point and end point; it is a circle of life. Birth and death are inexplicably linked; they are the same point at a gate to the final destination, our judgement at God's House. The paths we took determine the outcome after that.